THE VISCERA

Internal medicine in the era of ancient egyptians .

Dr.Alaaeldin Hamada

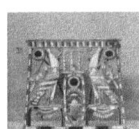

Copyright © 2021 Dr.Alaaeldin Hamada

All rights reserved

No part of this book may be reproduced, or stored in a retrieval system, or transmitted in any form or by any means, electronic, mechanical, photocopying, recording, or otherwise, without express written permission of the publisher.

ISBN: 9798494027399
Imprint: Independently published

Cover design by:
canopic jars
Library of Congress Control Number: 9798589752519
Printed in the United States of America

I dedicate this book to Imhotep "the great master ", and also my master who i never met but in his books ; Dr.Paul Ghalioungui .

CONTENTS

Title Page	1
Copyright	2
Dedication	3
Introduction	7
Preface	13
Prologue	15
CANOPIC JARS	19
INCANTATIONS	23
GENERAL INCANTATION	25
Okhdo	26
REMEDY	27
Edwin Smith Papyrus	29
hearst papyrus	81
berlin papyrus	92
ebers papyrus	117
REFRENCES	273
Afterword	283
Afterword	285
Books By This Author	287
Untitled	289

INTRODUCTION

The medicine of the ancient Egyptians is some of the oldest documented. From the beginnings of the civilization in the late fourth millennium BC until the Persian invasion of 525 BC, Egyptian medical practice went largely unchanged but was highly advanced for its time, including simple non-invasive surgery, setting of bones, dentistry, and an extensive set of pharmacopoeia. Egyptian medical thought influenced later traditions, including the Greeks.

Until the 19th century, the main sources of information about ancient Egyptian medicine were writings from later in antiquity. In 1822, the translation of the Rosetta stone finally allowed the translation of ancient Egyptian hieroglyphic inscriptions and papyri, including many related to medical matters (Egyptian medical papyri). The resultant interest in Egyptology in the 19th century led to the discovery of several sets of extensive ancient medical documents, including the Ebers papyrus, the Edwin Smith Papyrus, the Hearst Papyrus, the London Medical Papyrus and others dating back as far as 2900 BC.

The Edwin Smith Papyrus is a textbook on surgery and details anatomical observations and the "examination, diagnosis, treatment, and prognosis" of numerous ailments. It was probably written around 1600 BC, but is regarded as a copy of several earlier texts. Medical information in it dates from as early as 3000 BC. It is thus viewed as a learning manual. Treatments consisted of ointments made from animal, vegetable or fruit substances or minerals. There is evidence of oral surgery being performed as early as the 4th Dynasty (2900–2750 BC).

The Ebers papyrus (c. 1550 BC) includes 877 prescriptions – as categorized by a modern editor – for a variety of ailments and illnesses, some of them involving magical remedies, for Egyptian beliefs regarding magic and medicine were often intertwined. It also contains documentation revealing awareness of tumors, along with instructions on tumor removal.

The Kahun Gynaecological Papyrus treats women's complaints, including problems with conception. Thirty four cases detailing diagnosis and treatment survive, some of them fragmentarily. [Dating to 1800 BC, it is the oldest surviving medical text of any kind.

Other documents such as the Hearst papyrus (1450 BC), and Berlin Papyrus (1200 BC) also provide valuable insight into ancient Egyptian medicine.

Other information comes from the images that often adorn the walls of Egyptian tombs and the translation of the accompanying inscriptions. Advances in modern medical technology also contributed to the understanding of ancient Egyptian medicine. Paleopathologists were able to use X-Rays and later CAT Scans to view the bones and organs of mummies. Electron microscopes, mass spectrometry and various forensic techniques allowed scientists unique glimpses of the state of health in Egypt 4000 years ago.

The ancient Egyptians were at least partially aware of the importance of diet, both in balance and moderation. Owing to Egypt's great endowment of fertile land, food production was never a major issue, although, no matter how bountiful the land, paupers and starvation still exist. The main crops for most of ancient Egyptian history were emmer wheat and barley. Consumed in the form of loaves which were produced in a variety of types through baking and fermentation, with yeast greatly enriching the nutritional value of the product, one farmer's crop could support an estimated twenty adults. Barley was also used in beer. Vegetables and fruits of many types were widely grown. Oil was produced from the linseed plant and there was a limited selection of spices and herbs. Meat (sheep, goats, pigs) was regularly available to at least the upper classes and fish were widely consumed, although there is evidence of prohibitions during certain periods against certain types of animal products; Herodotus wrote of the pig as being 'unclean'. Offerings to King Unas (c. 2494–2345 BC) were recorded as "...milk, three kinds of beer, five kinds of wine, ten loaves, four of bread, ten of cakes four meats, different cuts, joints, roast, spleen, limb, breast, quail, goose, pigeon, figs, ten other fruits, three kinds of corn, barley, spelt, five kinds of oil, and fresh plants..."

It is clear that the Egyptian diet was not lacking for the upper classes and that even the lower classes may have had some selection (Nunn, 2002).

Like many civilizations in the past, the ancient Egyptians amply discovered the medicinal properties of plant life around them. In the Edwin Smith Papyrus there are many recipes to help heal different ailments. In a small section of this papyrus, there are five recipes one dealing with problems women may have had, three on techniques for refining the complexion, and the fifth recipe for ailments that deal with the colon. The ancient Egyptians were known to use honey as medicine, and the juices of pomegranates served as both an astringent and a delicacy. In the Ebers Papyrus, there are over 800 remedies; some were topical like ointments, and wrappings, others were oral medication such as pills and mouth rinses;still others were taken through inhalation.: The recipes to cure constipation consisted of berries from the castor oil tree, Male Palm, and Gengent beans, just to name a few. One recipe that was to help headaches called for "inner-of-onion, fruit-of-the-am-tree, natron, setseft-seeds, bone-of-the-sword-fish, cooked, redfish, cooked, skull-of-crayfish, cooked, honey, and abra-ointment.and 60 Some of the recommended treatments made use of cannabis and incense. Egyptian medicinal use of plants in antiquity is known to be extensive, with some 160 distinct plant products... Amidst the many plant extracts and fruits, the Egyptians also used animal feces and even some metals as treatments. These prescriptions of antiquity were measured out by volume, not weight, which makes their prescription making craft more like cooking than what Pharmacists do today.While their treatments and herbal remedies seem almost boundless, they still included incantations along with some therapeutic remedies.

Medical knowledge in ancient Egypt had an excellent reputation; while rulers of other empires would ask the Egyptian pharaoh to send them their best physician to treat their loved ones.[citation needed] Egyptians had some knowledge of human anatomy. For example, in the classic mummification process, mummifiers knew how to insert a long hooked implement through a nostril, breaking the thin bone of the braincase and removing the brain. They also had a general idea that inner organs are in the body cavity. They removed the organs through a small incision in the left groin. Whether this knowledge was passed down to the practitioners is unknown; yet it did not seem to have had any impact on their medical theories.

Egyptian physicians were aware of the existence of the pulse and its connection to the heart. The author of the Smith Papyrus even had a vague idea of the cardiac system. Although he did not know about blood circulation and deemed it unimportant to distinguish between blood vessels, tendons, and nerves. They developed their theory of "channels" that carried air, water, and blood to the body by analogies with the River Nile; if it became blocked, crops became unhealthy. They applied this principle to the body: If a person was unwell, they would use laxatives to unblock the "channels".

The oldest written text mentioning enemas is the Ebers Papyrus and many medications were administered using enemas. One of the many types of medical specialists was an Iri, the Shepherd of the Anus.

Many of their medical practices were effective, such as the surgical procedures given in the Edwin Smith papyrus. Mostly, the physicians' advice for staying healthy was to wash and shave the body, including under the arms, to prevent infections. They also advised patients to look after their diet, and avoid foods such as raw fish or other animals considered to be unclean.

PREFACE

here we are again with a new discovery extracted from ancient knowledge ; the gasrointestinal disases and treatment .this is the final honest translation from the original papyrus , moving from diffrent resources , original scripts , and liberaries .

the hardest problem for me is to recognising the substances names , eventhough it is confusing but in the end it is all about certain substances were used again and again .

maybe the diagnosis was not so clear because the symptoms were just mentioned in one line but now we have the knowledge about the substances connected with common gastroinetstinal diseases , therefore we can use these substances and make them part of our daily consumption .

PROLOGUE

Egyptian medical papyri are ancient Egyptian texts written on papyrus which permit a glimpse at medical procedures and practices in ancient Egypt. The papyri give details on disease, diagnosis, and remedies of disease, which include herbal remedies, surgery, and magical spells. It is thought there were more medical papyri, but many have been lost due to grave robbing. The largest study of the medical papyri to date has been undertaken by Berlin University and was titled Medizin der alten Ägypter ("Medicine of ancient Egypt").

Early Egyptian medicine was based mostly on a mixture of magic and religious spells. Most commonly "cured" by use of amulets or magical spells, the illnesses were thought to be caused by spiteful behavior or actions. Afterwards, doctors performed various medical treatments if necessary. The instructions for these medical rituals were later inscribed on papyrus scrolls by the priests performing the actions.

Main medical papyri:

Kahun Papyrus
Dated to circa 1800 BCE, the Kahun Gynaecological Papyrus is the oldest known medical text in Egypt. It was found at El-Lahun by Flinders Petrie in 1889, first translated by F. Ll. Griffith in 1893, and published in The Petrie Papyri: Hieratic Papyri from Kahun and Gurob. The papyrus contains 35 separate paragraphs relating to women's health, such as gynaecological diseases, fertility, pregnancy, and contraception. It does not describe sur-

gery.

Ramesseum Papyri :
The Ramesseum medical papyri consist of 17 individual papyri that were found in the great temple of the Ramesseum. They concentrate on the eyes, gynecology, paediatrics, muscles and tendons.

Edwin Smith Papyrus :
Dated to circa 1600 BCE, the Edwin Smith Papyrus is the only surviving copy of part of an ancient Egyptian textbook on trauma surgery. The papyrus takes its name from the Egyptian archaeologist Edwin Smith, who purchased it in the 1860s. The most detailed and sophisticated of the extant medical papyri, it is also the world's oldest surgical text. Written in the hieratic script of the ancient Egyptian language, it is thought to be based on material from a thousand years earlier.The document consists of 22 pages (17 pages on the recto, and 5 pages on the verso). 48 cases of trauma are examined, each with a description of the physical examination, diagnosis, treatment, and prognosis.An important aspect of the text is that it shows that the heart, liver, spleen, kidneys, ureters, and bladder were all known to the Egyptians, along with the fact that the blood vessels were connected to the heart. The entire translation is available online.

Ebers Papyrus
The Ebers Papyrus was also purchased by Edwin Smith in 1862. It takes its name from Georg Ebers who purchased the papyrus in 1872. The papyrus dates to around 1550BC and covers 110 pages, making it the lengthiest of the medical papyri. The papyrus covers many different topics including; dermatology, digestive diseases, traumatic diseases, dentistry and gynecological conditions. It makes many references to treating ailments with spells or religious techniques.[citation needed] One of the most important findings of this papyrus are the references to migraines which shows the condition dates back to this time.

Hearst Papyrus
The Hearst Papyrus was offered in 1901 to the Hearst Expedition in Egypt. It is dated around 2000 BC, though doubts subsist about its authenticity. It concentrated on treatments for problems dealing with the urinary system, blood, hair, and bites. It has been extensively studied since its publication in 1905.

London Papyrus:
The London Medical Papyrus is located in the British Museum and dates back to Tutankhamun. Although in poor condition, study of it has found it to focus on magical spells as remedy for disease.

Berlin Papyrus:
The Greater Berlin Papyrus, also known as the Brugsch Papyrus (Pap. Berl. 3038) was discovered by Giuseppe Passalacqua. It consists of 24 pages and is very similar to the Ebers Papyrus. Later sold to Friedrich Wilhelm IV of Prussia with other objects in 1827 for the Berlin Museum, the Greater Berlin Papyrus was translated into German in 1909.

Carlsberg Papyrus
The Carlsberg Papyrus is the property of the Carlsberg Foundation. The papyrus covers diseases of the eye and pregnancy.

Chester Beatty Medical Papyrus:
The Chester Beatty Medical Papyrus is named after Sir Alfred Chester Beatty who donated 19 papyri to the British Museum. The remedies in these texts are generally related to magic and focus on conditions that involve headaches and anorectal ailments.

Brooklyn Papyrus:
The Brooklyn Papyrus – Focusing mainly on snakebites, the Brooklyn Papyrus speaks of remedial methods for poisons ob-

tained from snakes, scorpions, and tarantulas. The Brooklyn Papyrus currently resides in the Brooklyn Museum

CANOPIC JARS

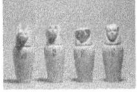

Canopic jars were used by the ancient Egyptians during the mummification process to store and preserve the viscera of their owner for the afterlife. They were commonly either carved from limestone or were made of pottery. These jars were used by the ancient Egyptians from the time of the Old Kingdom until the time of the Late Period or the Ptolemaic Period, by which time the viscera were simply wrapped and placed with the body. The viscera were not kept in a single canopic jar: each jar was reserved for specific organs. The term canopic reflects the mistaken association by early Egyptologists with the Greek legend of Canopus – the boat captain of Menelaus on the voyage to Troy – "who was buried at Canopus in the Delta where he was worshipped in the form of a jar". In alternative versions, the name derives from the location Canopus (now Abukir) in the western Nile Delta near Alexandria, where human-headed jars were worshipped as personifications of the god Osiris.

Canopic jars of the Old Kingdom were rarely inscribed and had a plain lid. In the Middle Kingdom inscriptions became more usual, and the lids were often in the form of human heads. By the Nineteenth Dynasty each of the four lids depicted one of the four sons of Horus, as guardians of the organs.

Use and design:
The canopic jars were four in number, each for the safekeeping of particular human organs: the stomach, intestines, lungs, and liver, all of which, it was believed, would be needed in the afterlife. There was no jar for the heart: the Egyptians believed it to be the seat of the soul, and so it was left inside the body.
These organs were removed from the body and carefully treated with natron (a natural preservative used by embalmers) and placed in the sacred Canopic Jars.

Many Old Kingdom canopic jars were found empty and damaged, even in undisturbed tombs. Therefore it seems that they were never used as containers. Instead, it seems that they were part of burial rituals and were placed after these rituals, empty
The design of canopic jars changed over time. The oldest date from the Eleventh or the Twelfth Dynasty, and are made of stone or wood. The last jars date from the New Kingdom. In the Old Kingdom the jars had plain lids, though by the First Intermediate Period jars with human heads (assumed to represent the dead) began to appear. Sometimes the covers of the jars were modeled after (or painted to resemble) the head of Anubis, the god of death and embalming. By the late Eighteenth Dynasty canopic jars had come to feature the four sons of Horus.Many sets of jars survive from this period, in alabaster, aragonite, calcareous stone, and blue or green glazed porcelain. The sons of Horus were also the gods of the cardinal compass points. Each god was responsible for protecting a particular organ and was himself protected by a companion goddess. They were:

- Hapi, the baboon-headed god representing the North, whose jar contained the lungs and was protected by the goddess Nephthys. Hapi is often used interchangeably with the Nile god Hapi, though they are actually different gods.

- Duamutef, the jackal-headed god representing the East, whose jar contained the stomach and was protected by the goddess Neith

- Imsety, the human-headed god representing the South, whose jar contained the liver and was protected by the goddess Isis

- Qebehsenuef, the falcon-headed god representing the West, whose jar contained the intestines and was protected by the goddess Serqet.

Early canopic jars were placed inside a canopic chest and buried in tombs together with the sarcophagus of the dead. Later, they were sometimes arranged in rows beneath the bier, or at the four corners of the chamber. After the early periods there were usually inscriptions on the outsides of the jars, sometimes quite long and complex. The scholar Sir Ernest Budge quoted an inscription from the Saïte or Ptolemaic period that begins: "Thy bread is to thee. Thy beer is to thee. Thou livest upon that on which Ra lives." Other inscriptions tell of purification in the afterlife.

In the Third Intermediate Period and later, dummy canopic jars were introduced. Improved embalming techniques allowed the viscera to remain in the body; the traditional jars remained a feature of tombs, but were no longer hollowed out for storage of the organs.

Copious jars were produced, and surviving examples of them can be seen in museums around the world.

In 2020, excavations at Saqqara showed that a woman called Didibastet, whose 2,600-year-old undisturbed tomb was discovered behind a stone wall, was entombed with six canopic jars instead of the traditional four. A CT scan revealed that the jars contain human tissue, suggesting that Didibastet's mummification was possibly the result of a specific request.

INCANTATIONS

magic spells

GENERAL INCANTATION

I -i.e: the doctor – graduated from the city of Ain Shams, With great warriors, lords of preservation and eternal rulers who protect me.
I came out from "sa el hagar" (ancient Egyptian city) with the mother of the gods to grant me their protection with my prayers.
I called upon the Almighty Lord to remove the divine headache (which is killing so much), this lord who exists In my head this and in my arms this and in my organs and in my hand this , to blame " sekhri " - the chief of diseases thunderbolts – for his enemies and his deputies.
The worshipped Thoth said a word and wrote it
And he composed a book that guides knowledge to scholars and those who know things, and to the wise, to serve him so that they may preserve the love of the deity who has given me life, because if he loves me he will give me life. "

This is said when a drug is administered to every affected organ, which saves a lot of protection.

OKHDO

Incantation for the Pain (Okhdo)

❝ The pain that comes out of (Beqet), which is not mentioned in the book that says: My arms reach the city of (Dedo) and weakens the city of (Dedt) , and that I ascend to the skies and see what happened there , and that nothing happened in the city (Al-Araba i.e : Abydos) to get over the divine aches And the agonizing pain, and the hurting pains, and the mortal pains, and the mortal headaches; that opens the mouth. And headaches from all things and diseases, which are in this body, in this flesh, and in these parts of my body.
The divine headaches, the cracked headaches, the crippled pain and the mortal pain are gone. As much as there are of every kind of bad headache in this flesh of my body, in this body and in these organs of mine..
I do not say nor do I repeat:"Wake up and vomit and perish as you happened."Say this four times and spit on the pain of human, as it has been tried thousands of thousands of times. "
Ebres 131

REMEDY

SYMPTOMS AND TREATMENT

EDWIN SMITH PAPYRUS

1500 BC

Definition of stomach pain:

If you examined a person whose stomach ache and eating bread makes him feel heavy, his stomach swollen and he is tired of walking ; like a person suffering from anal inflammation. Look at him while he is lying down, and if you find his stomach is hot and he is in pain from his stomach, tell him the medicine for the stomach:

By making for him the secret recipe, which is the weed that the doctor Ra made:
A plant called" Bakhti" and " date powder "
It is mixed and dipped in water and a person drinks it four mornings until his stomach is empty
And after you do that, if you find the two parts of his right stomach hot and the left cold, tell him that the disease is starting to come down what he ate, then repeat the examination for him, and you will find all his stomach is cold
Tell him that the intestines are relaxed i.e : they are released - and that the treatment has worked

Ebers 181

Dyspepsia :

If you examine a person whose stomach is in pain, and all of his organs are heavy, like a person who walks lethargy(in indo- lence), Put your hand on his stomach, and if you find it bloated and waving under your fingers, tell him that he has a glut
Do not order him to eat anything, but make him a purgative: the powder of soft dates, soften by sour beer, and he eats it as a bread.
And examine after that, and if you find his chest hot and his stomach cold, then say that this disease is gone, then order him

to protect his mouth from all harms.

Other :

If you examine a person who has a disease (i.e. flatulence) and he tends to vomit and that his droppings are on his side like a ball of stool (that is, stool) rising on his side and his stomach is distended
Make for him the original recipes for drinking, which are:
fresh bread grilled with oil and honey
ghathm (* most near world to it is thick milk) 1/32
And maidenhair fern 1/16
and myrrh (shasha) 1/8
By making it hot and mixed together for drinking in four days
If you examine him after that and find the disease mentioned in the previous description (his chest is hot and his stomach is cold), then he will be cured.

Other:

If you examine a person with pain in his stomach, and he is in pain in his arm, breast, and upper part of his stomach, say that he has sickness (i.e. a disease), and tell him that this is a symptom or death, or that the pain has subsided (i.e., it remained still), and make for him medicines prepared from grass:

acacia asak seeds 1
poppy 1
peppermint 1
aconitum (wolf'sbane)
Aegilops 1
Lindenbergia

Cook with oil and let the person drink it
Then put your hand on him, and if you find his elbow soft and his arm free of pain, tell him that the pain went down to the intestinal canal (and from it to the anus) and never repeat the treatment for him.

Other:

If you examine a person with epigastric pain and he is vomiting a lot, and you find him prominent at his stomach (from bloating) and his eyes are tired (i.e. sleepy) and his nose runs.
Tell him that this is one of the putrefactions of defecation, and that his excrement did not reach his buttocks, then do to him:
Wheat bread and ghazm (milk *)
 and add to them a cup of Haplophyllum tuberculatum and nutmeg, and he eats it hungry and eats fat beef and drinks a lot of beer until his eyes open and his nostrils clear and the faeces come down (that is, he defecates).

Other:

If you examine a person who has pain in his stomach, put your hand on him, and you will find that he is in pain with his spread vessels when placing fingers on him.
Tell him that this is fever (i.e inflammation) from pain in the spinal cord and give him weed medicines:

The red substance in soft wax is 5/6
Grilled in oil, honey and garlic 1/16
And Maidenhair fern 1/16
and myrrh 1/8
And the ground cyperus 1/16
And the aquatic cyperus 1/16
And wine and milk
The person eats it and drinks with it fresh beer until he recovers completely.

Other :

If you examine a person with a stomach disease and his arm,

breast, and half of his stomach are in pain, tell him that he is sick - i.e. a disease - and tell him that this is a symptom of the entry of death and that the disease has stayed (i.e. after its occurrence). Make weed medicines for him:

acacia asak seeds 1
poppy 1
peppermint 1
aconitum (wolf'sbane) 1
Aegilops 1
Lindenbergia seeds 1
Cook with beer and drink it
Then put your hand on him, and if you find his elbow soft and his forearm free from the disease, tell him that the disease went down to the intestines and to the anus, and never repeat the treatment for him.

N.B . " this prescription was mentioned before".

Other:

If you examine a person in pain during the day, like the man who ate dirty things and had a weak heart,
Tell him that death came from the accumulation of fecal matter and that it does not leave him, so he should not rely on weak treatment to not have a tumor and putrefaction.

Other :

If you examine a person with stomach pain, and his body is scrawny(weak) and totally lean .
If you examine him and do not find the disease in his entire stomach, rather you find him in a cleft of his stomach like a ball, tell him that you have danger.

And make him the following medicines:

Aswani grinded clay
 seed of a plant called (DSH)?
 colocynth cooked with oil and honey
A person eats it in four mornings until his thirst ends and his stomach pain goes away.

Other :

If you examine his stomach condition and find that its course is blocked and his stomach is distended and muffled, tell him that the blood has stopped and did not flow, and give him laxatives:

ghzm ? (milk) 1/8
Maidenhair fern 1/16
Terminalia 1/8
and myrrh (shasha) 1/8

To be cooked in a lot of beer and to be filtered it together and the person drinks it, then these droppings come out of his mouth or from his anus like pig's blood, and after that he warms up and covers it with a cover to moisten his stomach.

If you do not do this treatment for him, do for him an equal amount: of cow fat, turmeric seed, (NS) ?, myrrh and thistle.
It is cooked and painted .

Other:

If you examine a sick person with pain in the mouth of his stomach, and you find the mouth of his stomach is waving under your fingers like oil inside the bag, tell him that it will come out of his mouth like urine and do to him:

doum 5/6

Date flour(powder) 5/6

mix them , knead them in male urine, then mash them and cook them with oil and honey, and the person eats them in four mornings,

and add on this grain called (Maqat) hot and grinded.

Other :

If you examine a sick person with epigastric pain , and you find on his back like loads of KHRT ? (KHRT is the bumps: ? : a disease that weakens the body and makes the milk of the animal flow), then tell him that it was a prick in his back and that it affectet his back and caused pain to it . and make for him the back treatment to enter him and get through him .
and make to him KHMT and give him back treatment which is :
Qat 1
peppermint 1
acacia leaf 1
mud from wall 1
It is grinded and cooked and with beer scum and paint for four days until it heals quickly.

Other :

If you examine a person with stomach ache and find him very disoriented, tell him that this pain befell you like a fit that touched your body (i.e bad spirit)

And make for him :
garlic 1
myrrh 1
cyperus from sea (1
ground cyperus 1
And colocynth
By cooking with a fresh beer , this remedy removes pain.

Other :

If you examine a person with a stomach disease and he vomits and suffers a lot and ache like a person with a groin (yellowing with a swelling in the face), tell him that he had a prick tighten on him and make him a dose, which is:
fig 1/8
Milk 1/16
flour 1/8
kept allover night with ½ . fresh beer

filter it and drink a lot of it to recover quickly.

Other:

If you examine a person who is in pain in his stomach, and you find his right side tense, say that he suffered from a prick which turned to swelling, and make for him the current medicines, which are:
Doum ;
filter and drink for four days.

If you examine him after this work and find that his diseases remain as they were before, make for him the appropriate medicines until the disease is removed and cured, which are:
Acacia asak seeds 1/64
And a handful of salt grind together and cook with fresh beer fresh
then make the appropriate medicines for him with oil to make it

go (that is, to remove the pain) which is :
Lindenbergia that is cooked with oil and honey and a person eats it for four days.

Other :

A)
If you examine a person who is in pain on his left side and his leg joint is unable to walk on the ground,
Tell him: Go to the coast and cover yourself with sand
And do the previous treatment:
grated lemon 1/4
garlic 1/8
Maidenhair fern 1/16
Cook one thing in 2/3 . oil
and honey 1/3
And a person eats it in four days.

B)
If you examine a person after this work and find him walking and jogging in the open, make for him a plant called "Tamw" ? and a "FSEET " ?.(N.B : in arabic dictionary its part in date fruit between the funnel and the kernel of dates"
They are cooked properly and a person eats them until he fills his stomach and fills his gut for four days.
Then put your hand on it, and if you find the sicknes is cut and

crushed as wheat is crushed: do the cooling for it immediately, which is:
Doum or seed called (OAH)? 1 and water
Filter and eat in four days.

Other:

A)

If you examine a person who is sick with his stomach and find that he has diarrhea and was in pain next to his stomach, and it was smothering (i.e. not draining) bread, and it was heavy as if a worm (patu)? had entered it, then strive with him with the appropriate medicines by taking barley water..
If the stomach moves under your fingers:

B)

Do this to him four mornings, and he will obtain the necessary constipation on his own (and originally from itself, the medicine enters him, i.e. the necessary blockage).
and make for him :
Carob 1/3
and gum grip 1/8
And lead rust 1/16
That it be cooked with oil and honey and eaten in four days

C)

Then after that go through your fingers. If you find the stomach is like grain of sand and all the parts are hot, and the bread is fermenting in it and scattered like the clay bread inside its stomach, then it becomes easy(gets out with stool).

Other:

If you examine a person whose stomach is in pain, and his stomach is mobbed and in pain, and all the bread that entered it with food fermented in his stomach, and he was in pain in his legs and the soles of his feet, not his feet.

If you examine him and find that his stomach is clogged like a woman who beat a boy (with effort) and she became humiliated (meaning lean) for this reason,

Tell him the repellent drugs according to the decision of the wiseman "i.e the doctor ", who does not exclude your sister herself, which is:
dry green barley, cook it in water and do not make it evaporate, take it out of the fire and mix it with date flour.
Then it is filtered and eaten in four days until the person recovers.

Other :

A)

If you examine a person who has stomach disease, and he has a mob in his stomach, and his face is yellow, and the mouth of his stomach is blocked, then examine him.
You find his stomach is inflamed and his abdomen is stretched

Know that it is the latent heat and that the inflammation consumes it (that is, exhausts it).

B)

Make for him a medicine to cool the infections, to loosen his gut, by drinking fresh beer with "shweet"? flour, so he eats from it and drinks for four days.

And that it be in the morning every day until it comes out of his anus (i.e. it eases), and if the stool comes down like black seeds (naazto ? maybethe goat), tell him that this infection came down from his stomach and the stinking solidation that was in his stomach has gone away.

C)

If you examine him after this work, and the substances are coming down from his anus like beans, and they are soggy at the time of ejaculation, like the starch of fodder (ie, sandy bread), tell him that what was in his stomach is gone

And make him cool medicines by putting the pot on the fire and he will sweat with a suitable temperature (i.e. he will sweat with steam).

Another Remedy For Stomach Disease:

buckthorn bread 1
watermelon 1
cat shit 1
fresh beer 1
wine 1
Make one thing and put it on it.

Others To Treat The Right Side And Remove Nso ? (Upset):

(shnf)? 1
white Lindenbergia 1/8
green Lindenbergia 1/8
poppy fiber 1/16
Juniper seeds 1/16
field turmeric 1/8
water trumeric 1/8 ?
iris 1/8
myrrh 1/16
Qat 1/8
green painting substance 1/8
Civet 1/16
Cistanche tubulosa 1/8
honey 1/32
beer 1/3
goose fat 1/8

It is kept in the dew, filtered and is eaten in four days.

Other: To Remove Pain From The Right Side When It Is Severe With Inflammation:

fig 1/8
Terminalia 1/8
frankinsence 1/8
white pastry 1/32
flour 1/16
Lead Rust 1/32
acacia leaff 1/32
wine 1/3
buckthorn leaf 1/32
Sycamore leaf 1/32
beer 1/3 dana
It is kept in the dew, is filtered and eaten in four days.

Other: To Remove The Pain That Consumes (Ie, Debilitating) Stomach Blood:

A type of beer called (Tanshpet)? 1
raw dough 1
Faaq (cooked oil) 1
Make one thing and put it on it.

Another Treatment For The Stomach:

carob 1/3
Black nightshade 1/3
(SNDH)? (most close word is sandi :pomelo) 1/4
a little fig
Sycamore flour or colocynth (bitter melon) from oasis
It is finely grinded and placed on a fresh beer of good wheat, and it remains in the dew without seeing the dryness or covering it. then put honey 1/3 and goose fat and mix together and drink it by the man or the woman .

Other: To Remove Stomach Disease:

buckthorn bread 1
cat poop 1
lead oxide 1
watermelon 1
fresh beer 1

wine 1
Mix it together and put it on.

Another Treatment For The Stomach:

honey 1
Faaq (cooked oil) 1
Frankinsence 1
wine 1
Mixed together, cooked and eaten.

Other :

honey 2
Doum powder 2
SNDH ? 1
Four tablets are made over four days by first cooking honey, then dropping the doUm and SNDH* powder on it and eat it in four days.

Other For The Stomach:

Frankinsence 1/64
Maidenhair fern 1/3
SINDH* 1/4
honey ¼
wine 1/3
goose fat 1/3
Cook and eat in one day .

Starting Antiemetics:

green colocynth
It is placed on water in new pot and a person drinks it in four days.

Other:

colocynth cooked with fresh beer and drink a third of it in four days .

Other :

Take an amount of (Min) one, half of which is water, and half of it colocynth, and keep it for four days exposed to the sun and overnight, and make it increase by 1/12 of this (Min).
And let the one who vomits drink it for four days, and he will recover immediately.

N.b: Min is a measurement unit .

Other:

one HNW of the date flour who makes a dough and put it in two clay pots, and this dough stays in them until it cracks.
After that, bsisa is made with fat and a person eats it hot, so he becomes fine and heals immediately.

N.b: Hnw is a measurement unit
n.b2: Bsisa is a typical Mediterranean food, based on flour of roasted barley , a variety of mixtures of roasted cereals ground with fenugreek and aniseed and cumin and sugar

Other :

Boiled cow's milk, then bring the fresh dates (ma'hout, in Arabic, maho) mixed and put milk cream on it.
A person eat all and drink hot milk for four days.

Other :

Date flour is placed in a bag of cloth,
And make this bundle in honey for a day
Then put it on the fire until the dough cracks.
This preserved packet is placed in a pot and water is placed on it

and filtered (like making beer) and it is eaten for four days.

Other :

fermenting dough 1/4
oil 1/4
beer 1/4
Placed in boiler and cooked and then dished with (AWF?) 1 and khat 1
It is placed in this boiler and served to be cooked, filtered and given to drink for four days.

Other :

Date flour 1/3
Put it on water and make leaven (let it ferment) and water it .
Put two pots on the fire to heat it, then put this yeast in them and make it a dough. When it is cooked, make it bsissa with honey and cow fat to be eaten in one day.

Other :

Cow's milk and carob are placed in pot that are put on fire as beans are roasted. After roasting, the person chews the carob and drinks this milk for four days.

Other :

Honey and cream make one thing, and the patient eats it, drinks beer, and eats Salvadora persica for four days.

Other:

A pig tooth , finely grinded and placed in four tablets and eaten for four days .

Other :

SIRAM? water
Bread
 cream
grilled and is eaten with a pie for four days.

N.B : siram is date or palm piece.

Other:

Doum powder 1/3
goose fat 1/3
honey 1/3
Cook and eat for four days.

Other :

Date powder 1/32
SHNF? 1/32
garlic 1/8
SNDH ? 1/8

It is finely ground and mixed together and placed on a DNH"dja" of beer, then overnighted outdoor , filtered and eaten within four days.

N.B :Dja   dja   0.30 L .

Other :

garlic 1/32
Ameem? 1/32
Finely grinded and put it on the fire and smoke its steam by reed for one day.

To Remove Vomit From The Stomach:

fig 1/8
Terminalia (Tropical almond) 1/8
Black nightshade 1/16

cumin 1/64
acacia paper 1/32
MIDAD (ink ?) 1/64
Peppermint 1/32
hop 1/8
fresh beer 1.

kept outdoor and eaten for four days.

Other:

Roasted doum, brewed in hot beer in a "BATYA " i.e :pot made of wood , and make a bread that is eaten for two days.

Other :

honey 1 HNW *
cow fat 1 MD*
Water and SIRAM W MD*
Doum roasted 1 MD *
acacia ash.
grinded as one thing , cooked and eaten hot with a finger.

N.B :
HNW:an old measure : Jar :   0.48 L
MD : an old measure : 1/2 cup
SIRAM : date or palm piece.

Other :

colocynth fresh is placed in a pot , half of which are water, and half of which are a colocynth , and drink from it here every day for four days .

Other:

The seeds of Euphorbia helioscopia "i.e : the sun spurge " 1
wax 1
mixed as one thing
Bring seven stones and heat them in the fire and take one of them and put this medicine on it and cover it in a new pot and pierce the bottom of it and put your mouth in a reed and suck out the steam that is in it and do this with all the remaining stones . "smoke it "
then eat fatty food after that like fat meat or fat.

The Principle Of Drugs For The Treatment Of The Liver:

fig 1/8
Medicinal fruits? 1/8
grape raisin 1/16
flour 1/8
poppy 1/16
soggy 1/32
frankinsence 1/64
SHMT ? * 1/64
water 5/6
It is kept outdoor , filtered, and a person eats it for four days.

N.B: SHMT : most common translation is white hair .

Other :

fig 1/8
Black nightshade 1/8
Maidenhair fern 1/16
Myrtus communis 1/16
frankinsence 1/16
Lead Rust 1/32
water 1/32
it is kept outdoor, filtered, and a person eats it for days.

Other :

lotus blossom 1/8
DNH* from the West (i.e. wine)
Buckthorn flour 1/8
fig 1/8
Milk 1/16
Juniper seeds 1/16
Frankinsence 1/64
A handful (DNH)* of fresh beer kept outdoor , filtered and eaten for four days.

N.B: DNH is a measure .

Other :

fig 1/8
fruit ? 1/8
ANOSI * (Salvia aegyptiaca) 1/4
buckthorn bread 1/8
colocynth 1/32
flour 1/16
grape raisin 1/8
SHMT ** 1/64
Frankinsence 1/64
A handful of fresh beer kept outside, filtered and eaten for four days.

Other :

fig 1/8
flour 1/8
Juniper seeds 1/16
southern Natroun " from upper egypt " 1/8
One dna of water, kept outdoor, filtered and eaten for four days.

Starting Medicines To Treat The Right Side Of Stomach From Writhing In Pain(Stomach Ache And Distortions):

fresh bread 1/32
skhetite ? * syrup 1/32
ghee

……… is placed on it.

N.B: skhtite is : pure white flour , the syrup maybe its meant beer.

Other :

Frankinsence 1/64
Juniper seeds 1/16
Adenosma 1/16
Abeqa? 1/16
Turmeric from mountain 1/16
turmeric from sea 1/16
Linseed 1/16
garlic 1/16
fine linen 1/16
qabaa? 1/16
stah ? 1/16
white small pearls 1/16
fresh small pearls 1/16
goose fat 1/3
Cyperus (Nutsedges) 1/16

doum 1/3
Aswan clay 1/16
Qat 1/8
honey 1/32

bind .

N.B: in berlin papyrus comes with very old names .

Other :

Fennel
Black nightshade 1
doum 1
bread 1
HMAMI? 1
Cassia fistula 1
Barley seeds 1

Mix it together and poultice* it.

N.B: A poultice, also called a cataplasm, is a soft moist mass, often heated and medicated, that is spread on cloth and placed over the skin to treat an aching, inflamed or painful part of the body. It can be used on wounds such as cuts.
'Poultice' may also refer to a porous solid filled with solvent used to remove stains from porous stone such as marble or granite.

Other :

cyperus (nutsedges) 1
goose fat 1
honey 1

poultice .

HEARST PAPYRUS

2nd millennium BC

For abdominal diarrhea*:
Myrrh 1/32
Mix it with well water and make 7 pills and mix it with honey and the patient takes it .

N.B:
to induce diarrha and cleaning the stomach .

Another Recipe For Diarrhea:

A handful of table salt mixed with honey
A person drinks it and then eats a little honey on his finger and

then drinks fresh beer for four days.

A Recipe For Painful Anal Disease:

Khat ,
placed on it.

For A Sore Anus:

Warmed by stone, sand or fresh beer scum.

Treatment Of The Left Side Of The Abdomen:

seeds of plant is called in ancient Egyptian (khadab) and in Arabic, "khadab" ¼
Cordia myxa 1/8
black nightshade 1/8
Anusi? (anis ?) 1
gum 1/32
Lead Rust 1/32
Frankinsence 1/62
 1/62
latency
Pure (sour plant) water

it is kept all night in the dew, then filtered and is eaten for four days

Note from the author:
Pain in the left abdomen is common in Irritable Bowel Syndrome

The Treatment Of The Disease Called (Sah'et)

which is equivalent to it in Arabic, which is a tumor in the abdomen under the diaphragm:

Sycamore milk and colocynth powder are placed on it.

Stomach Disease Treatment:

Date powder ¼
colocynth 1/32
A plant like barley? 1/3
fresh beer
Ameem? 1/3

It is filtered and the patient eats it over four days after dividing into parts, each part equals 1/2 tnat .

Another Treatment:

milk 1/3
honey 1/14
water 1/2 tnat

Cooked and filtered and eaten for four days.

Medicine To Keep Food In The Stomach (I.e. To

Prevent Vomiting):

fig 1/8
Anusi (salvia agyptiaga) 1/8
Lead Rust 1/32
honey 1/32
Water 1/3 tinat .

Cooked and filtered and eaten for four days.

Bowel Treatment:

Lead Rust 1/32
gum 1/32
honey 1/8
fig 1/8

1 tinat water

It is kept outdoor and is eaten for four days.

For Abdominal Diarrhea:

milk 1/3
NAKAWY? ¼
honey ¼

Cooked and filtered and eaten for four days.

To Remove Vomiting:

milk 1/3
AM? 1/16
Karaj (moldy bread) 1/16
frankinsence 1/64
A plant called (hay) 1/8

Cook and eat for four days.

Abdominal Diarrhea Treatment:

1/3 . donkey milk
acacia paper 1/16
Indigo (Indigofera) 1/16
A plant called Duat 1/32
Juniper powder 1/16
honey 1/16

It is cooked, filtered and used by the patient for four days.

BERLIN PAPYRUS

1200 BC.

Treatment of vomiting:
Fresh morning cow mik cream and honey that a person eats for four days.

Another Remedy To Ward Off Vomiting In Children:

dry dates
wheat groats.

grinded softly on HN * of milk and the patient drinks it.

N.B:
hn is a measure.

To Ward Off Vomiting:

milk cream
cumin

Mixed with honey and eaten for four days.

Other :

Shenf ? 1/16
Acacia Asak 1/16
ghzm ? 1/8
dough ¼

As before (mixed and eaten for four days).

Other:

¼ . gum
honey ¼

Cooked and a person drink it .

Other :

Siram (the rest of milk after udder drying)* ½
honey 1/3
cream 1/3

Mix it together and the patient takes it for four days.

N.B: siram is a process after milking is the rest of milk inside animal breast .

Other To Silence Vomiting:

Auf?* 1
fresh beer 1
fat 1
Qat 1
A water called (Away) 1

Mixed together (and taken) over four days.

N.b:
auf has many translations ,most close is a plant with good smell

To Improve Vomiting Bout(State):

colocynth 1/16
Grape 1/3
gum 1/32
honey 1/8

Mixed together and taken for four days.

Others (In Order To Improve Nausea) And Vomiting:

Milk
cream
A drink called "Mahalot" that the patient drinks for four days.

Other :

wine
lake salt

It is finely grinded and used by the patient for four days.

Other :

acacia leaf
honey
fresh beer

The patient drinks it.

Other :

cream
cumin

the patient eats.

Other :

Pig fat 1/3
Sweeda (i.e wheat) 1/3
goose fat 1/3

It is kept in the dew for four days and is used by a man or a woman infected with a burn*.

N.B:
burn is meant mainly to be heartburn, acidity, GERD.

Other :

colocynth water
honey

eaten.

Another Remedy To Ward Off Vomiting:

shnf?
Acacia asak
ghzm?
hasa*?

It is cooked and used by the patient for four days

N.B:
Hasa: a delicate food made from flour and water.

Other :

colocynth
yamqor ?* from the seashore
suwaiq ?**

It is grinded soft and eaten by a person, it's tried (i.e : guranteed).

N.B:
yaqmor is something bitter
suwaiq is grinded wheat and barley

Other:

waban?

myrhh

grinded with ghazm? and made as seven tablets (grains) And they are placed in a bowl with a cover , and a pot with a reed inside this pot , and half of it is placed in the person's mouth, so he can swallow(smoke) it and see if the person is vomiting .

N.B:
obviously it is a primitive way to make a water pipe(hookah)

To Relieve Vomiting:

cream
cumin

They are mixed with honey and eaten by the patient for four days.

Stomach Pain Treatment:

Anib (eggplant?)
Black nightshade (qanat)?*
sycamore powder
Aswan clay
wax
carob

Human is exposed to the somke of it. "insence"

N.B:
maybe it is tnat " a measure "

Others For Stomach Pain:

sea salt
Fresh(dulcet) beer scum

insence him . "i.e :expose the erson to the smoke "

Acute Gastroesophageal Reflux Disease (Sach N Hp Tau):

Symptoms of the disease :
The patient's body is heavy

And the mouth of his stomach hurts, and his stomach hurts and low .
And his clothes weigh him down
And his many clothes do not warm him
And thirsty at night
And his stomach tastes like fog, like a person who ate sycamore
And his flesh is as dead as a man who walked a lot on the road
If he sits to defecate, his anus is heavy and does not come out
Tell him :
He has gasterointeritis in the center of prickles .
And that his heart is aching, and hurts if it moves, make for him the prescriptions of taking the first time to remove the prickling from his body.
Carob grinded with water 1/3
fresh bread 1/8
fresh dates ¼
And juniper seeds 1/16
A plant called (Trent)? 1/32
and honey 1/16
and milk 1/8
And Cyperus rotundus (nut grass) 1/8
A liquid called (Ayaat)? ½
It is finely grinded and poultice it.

Other:

live meat ¼
lemon 1/8
Aconitum(wolf's bane) 1/8
am? 1/16
Juniper seeds 1/32
sutah? 1/16
Cyperus rotundus (nut grass) 1/32
1/8 . grape
1/8 . hay
frankinsence 1/64

Shanf ? (a plant that is said to be lasq)
lantanas
 Dates 1/32
goose fat 1/8
Fresh beer 5/6

It is finely grinded and filtered, and the patient takes it for four days

Other :

Agnes(sndh)? 1/8
honey 1/8
1/3 . fresh beer

The patient drinks it for four days.

To Remove The Satiety That Weighs The Abdomen (Ie, Satiety And Indigestion):

I make for him recipes that repel stomach pain and keep the prickles away:
fig 1/8
Cyperus rotundus (nut grass) 1/8
grape 1/8
Juniper seeds 1/16
sutah? 1/32
fuseet ?* 1/8
Aconitum 1/8
Naqawy? ¼
Frankinsence 1/64
Auf? 1/8
turmeric from mountain 1/8
turmeric from water 1/32
fresh bread 1/8
lean meat any fat 1/3

amem? 5/6
goose fat 1/8
Fresh beer 5/6

It is mixed, filtered, and eaten by the patient for four days.

N.B:
fuseet :date Perianth

Treatment For A Person With Stomach Pain:

Make him the first recipe for removing the prickles from his body:
am?1/8
Cyperus rotundus (nut grass) 1/8
goose fat 1/8
Fresh beer 5/6

It is finely grinded, filtered, and drunk by the patient for four days

Other:

Cyperus rotundus (nut grass) 1/8
fig 1/8
sutah? 1/8
Fresh beer 5/6

It is cooked and drunk by a person with this disease

Other:

Faaq? (cooked oil) 1/8
honey 1/8
buckthorn leaf 1/8
acacia leaf 1/8
kht leaf 1/8

kept in the dew, gets beaten (mixed) with water and injected into the anus in one day.

Incantation:

"I am the idol of Horus
Son of the god Asuris
in Saraya
I'm coming to see what happens.
Healing comes useful in peace from...... on my right"

This is said while mixing the substances

With water, the patient drinks it and recovers immediately.

EBERS PAPYRUS

1550 BC

Treatment to loosen the abdomen (that is, to release it):
Milk ½ dna
¼ . flour
honey ¼

Cooked, filtered and eaten in four days.

Another Treatment For Abdominal Dislocation, I.e. Releasing It:

seeds of plant called (Wam)?* 1

eggplant 1
Monotropa seeds 1
honey 1
Shanf (a plant called paste)?

Mixed together and eaten by humans in four days.

Other:

garlic 1
colocynth (start to be yellow) 1
cumin 1
fig 1
Fruit (one of the fruits used in medicine)
wolf's bane (black nightshade) 1
fat 1

Mixed together and eaten by humans.

Other: To Empty The Abdomen (That Is, To Empty It Of Fecal Matter):

cow milk 1
flour 1
honey 1

It is kneaded softly and cooked and eaten in one day.

Other For The Abdomen:

Parts of the castor tree ¼
Bernie (i.e:the finest dates)
 thifat? (i.e: mustard) 5/6
cyperus (nutsedges) 1/16
Poppy root 1/16
coriander 1/16
Beer and a drink called (Bajt)

It is kept in the dew, filterED and is eaten in four days.

Others: To Remove Flatulence (And It Is Called In Egyptian Warmy I.e Tumor)

black nightshade 1

It is cooked in cow's milk or in fresh beer, and the person drinks it to remove the bloating from his stomach.

Others: For Stomach Diarrhea And To Remove All The Bad Things In The Human Body:

sindh? 1/8
honey 1/8
Bernie (the best of date fruits) 1/3
carob 1/3

Mix together and drink in one day.

Another Recipe:

dough 1/2
ghzm ?1/32
am (grass) 1/32
garlic 1/32
Prostrate knotweed 1/16
cyperus(nutsedges) 1/32
Juniper seeds 1/16
Frankinsence 1/64
sea salt 1/32
Divide into 5/6

And honey is poured on it Consecutively and taken from the fire after it is shortened to the size of a finger, and it is drunk on a day.

Another Treatment For The Stomach:

sindah 1/4
hop

¼ ghzm ?(vegetable acid)
Fresh beer 5/6

Mixed together, cooked, filtered and eaten in one day, it facilitates the human being and removes all the faeces present in the abdomen.

Other:for Diarrhea In The Stomach And Expelling Faeces From The Human Stomach:

Castor bean is chewed and drunk with beer, and all that is in the stomach will come out.

Treatment, Which Is The Third Prescription For Defecation:

honey 1
yrrh (shasha) 1
ghzm? 1
prostorate knotweed 1
Juniper berries 1
Heart of a plant (azit)? 1
cumin 1
seeds of am? (grass?) 1

garlic 1
sea salt 1

Make a pill and put it in the anus.

To Fix Urine And Facilitate Defecation:

1/3 . goose fat
colocynth 1/32

Cook and boil until it is shortened to a finger and drink with wine.

Other To Facilitate Defecation:

hop 1/6 (which is like the Phoenician bean)
Corchorus olitorius seeds
mixed with a sindah

grind it it finely and put it on honey and drink it with date wine 1/3.

Other:

Prostrate knotweed 1/8
honey 1/8

Cook and boil until shortened to a finger and drink with frothy beer mix in one day.

Others: To Ward Off Painful Stools In The Human Stomach:

White bread (discorides de mal.)
Red grains called (Nabt)? 1
woman's milk

Mix it together and drink it.

Other:

wheat flour 1
garlic 1
Juniper beans 1
Prostrate knotweed 1
hop 1
Lindenbergia 1

It is cooked together and made into bread and eaten by a person.

Other: For Abdominal Diarrhea And Defecation (Ie, Cleaning The Stomach)

Fist of Rumex vesicarius seeds

It is finely grinded and placed in four loaves, mixed with honey, and eaten by humans.

Other:

Pigment (or iron filings?) which is green dye 1/64
honey
same , as before.

Treatment For Releasing Abdomen (Emptying It):

sindah? 1
Prostrate knotweed 1
goose fat 1
honey 1
fresh beer

it is made one thing (ie mixe together) and drink in four days.

Other To Ward Off All Diseases Of The Abdomen And To Treat The Intestines? Or Lung:

Frothy fresh beer
colocynth 1/2

Put it in a bowl and use it as an ointment against the disease of death and knead with foam and boil it every time you want to use it.

For Abdominal Diarrhea (And In The Original To Make The Abdomen Escape From The Najw?*):

Fresh beer 1/3 dna
Shanf (a plant called paste or rabbit's ear) 1/1
sea salt 1/16
And a fruit (of fruits used medically) 1/8

Soften with water and drink in four days

N.B:
An-Naju: What comes out of the stomach of gases and faeces

Other:

Hino* dried and toasted barley 1 , make it bread
Fat is added to it and a person eats it, then survives.

To Repair The Guts:

Myrrh called Shasha 1
sunflower (Helianthus) 1
charcoal 1
Pigment part
honey 1

Eat before bed.

Other:

Roasted figs mixed with fresh faq(cookedoil)
 and black nightshades.

Hanu* from Fayhaa (food made from flour and water in addition to spices, and we considered that the heart sign written in Egyptian reads "Ah")*
Food that corresponds to the Egyptian Bahi
Mixes together and eaten by the patient with abdominal pain.

Other: To Remove Abdominal Disease:

oil

carob
ghzm?
Wheat

It is cooked in honey and mixed together and eaten in one day.

For Constipation (Ie Retention Of Stool):

fresh lamp 1/8
fresh bread 1
oil 1
honey ¼
wax 1/16
Water 1/3 DNA

It is settled and eaten in four days.

Other:

bread pulp 1/11
Lead Rust 1/32
Abtandoa* Drink 1/16
Water 1/3 DNA
It is eaten in four days.

* Abtandoa: a compound word from two words, the first abt and designated with a round sign, and the second is the name of a vessel topped by the fold, i.e. the parable, and it is a common word in the general custom.
OVUM SIRE GLOBULUS

Other:

shnaf? 1/8
fruit called ASHAD? 1/8
Black nightshade 1/16
Salvia aegyptiaca 1/16
Juniper beans 1/66
honey 1/16
water 1/3

It is quenched with water (i.e. irrigated) and eaten within four days.

Other:

Bread pulp (chuns) 1/16
Syrup (Abtendo) 1/8
coloynth 1/32
water 1/3

Drink in four days.

Other:

fig 1/8
grape 1/8
flour 1/32
soggy 1/32
Lead Rust 1/64
colocynth 1/32
Maidenhair fern 1/8

Then repeat:

    "o donkey

    o female donkey" .. repeat

    "o Azn

    O Aznit" .. repeat

It is mixed with water and the patient takes it for four days.

Other:

To cut stools accompanied by a lot of blood (hemorrhoids)? :
fresh dates 1/8
crushed carob 1/3
fat 1/8
honey 1/8

Filter and eat in four days.
Each treatment is the same as a second (i.e. the two treatments before each other)

To Kill The Worm (Haft), In Arabic, Haft, Ascaris Lumbricoides

Pomegranate peel 1/3
water 1/2
Mixed with water, filtered and eaten in one day.

Other:

Saidi* barley 1/3

sea salt 5/6
water 1/2

Mixed with water, filtered and eaten in one day.

N.B:
saidi : from upper egypt

Other

acacia leaves 1/3
water 1/2

Mixed with water, filtered and eaten in one day.

To Remove The Worm (Heft) From The Abdomen:

Pigment (green dye) 4 pieces made into four loaves and used by humans.

Other:

Hatata (heart) Monotropa 1/3
siram? 1/3
½ . water
1/3 yaqno (i.e. mixed with water)

And filtered and eaten in one day.

To Kill The Worm (Heft)

Date powder 1/8
colocynth 1/8
fresh beer 1/3

Cook, filter and eat.

Other:

twigs of coriander (vegetable) 1/3
ghzm? 1/3
Fresh beer 1 dna

It is cooked, pressed, and eaten.

Other:

Ht (heart) of Monotropa,
It is placed inside a khimt? for four days and irrigated with water and squeezed into five (or 1/5) containers which is good for the ear if it is not black, and water is added to it in the summer and drunk in the morning.

Other:

cyperus (cyperus tuber forme)?* 1/32
pigment? (green dye) or iron filings 1/32
water 1/3

Cook and eat in four days.

N.B:
In Egypt, tiger nuts are known by the name Hab el-Aziz and after softening it by soaking in water, it is sold on hand carts as a street food.[19] Its popularity was depicted in movies, such as the song named after it:

Other:

A beans called (Wam)? ¼
Shenf? ¼

Hat (heart) of Monotropa 1/8
honey 1/8
beer 1/3

It is grinded and mixed with honey, and in the morning it is added to 1/3 of the beer and eaten.

Other:

beans called (Wam)? 1/3
2/3 . water
It is irrigated with water and drink or beer added to it.

Other:

Myrtus 1/3
sunflower ¼
Cooked with honey and eaten.

> "They recite an incantation , so people will get rid of,and will be saved from : weakness .and worms will be removed from my stomach. And the idol did what the enemy did. So he enchanted and undid what had happened to my somach ." *

N.B:
incantation

Other: A Useful Stomach Medicine:

Myrtus 1
sunflower 1

It is finely grinded and cooked in honey and eaten by a person who has worms in his stomach, because worms are the cause of AIA: sickness (that is, weakness) that is fatal against every medicine.

Other:

Pomegranate peel mixed with beer 1/3
And it is watered in a bowl of 5/6 of water
And in the morning with a rag and a person drinks it.

Haft : Ascaris Lumbricoides

Auf ? 1
sghm
ghzm
dough 1

mix together and eat , defecate all the worms in the stomach .

The Treatment Of The Worm Haft (And In Arabic Haft):

Dry sycamore fruits 1
dates 1
and strong beer 1

mix well and put on strong beer and the person drink it.

To Ward Off The Pain Caused By The Snake, Haft And The Worm Bind:

Dom powder 1
Shawshi Al-Ameem ? 1
goose fat 1

Mixed together, filtered and eaten in four days

To Ward Off The Pain Caused By The Worm. Bnd:

acacia leaf 1
Leaves or branches of peppermint? 1 auf? 1
A plant called (Sas)? 1

Mix one thing and put it on the stomach of a woman or a man.

A Treatment To Kill The Worm (Haft), Which Is One Of The Belly Snakes:

Acacia leaves are placed on water in container and covered with a rag.
In the day, Put in Hon* from stone and grind it then put in a ...... with a linen and then drink it (this was mentioned like that)

N.B:

hon : is a grinder

Other:to Remove The Disease Causing The Worm (Bind) T.mediocancllata

black nightshade 1
anp? (eggplant) 1
linen oqd? (necklace or knot) 1
honey 1

dose in four days.

To Kill The Snake Named (Haft) And In Arabic Al-Haffath (Which Is One Of The Belly Snakes)

seeds of plant called (Wam)? 18
Shenf? 1/16
sea salt 1/32
honey 1/8

make one thing and drink in one day.

Another Treatment:

dry Sycamore 1
Fresh dates 1
grinded in beer 1
And drink in four days.

Bnd (To Kill The Worm Bnd)

Hat (heart) of Monotropa 1/3
corn 1 dna

Cook, filter and eat immediately.

Other :

grains of plant called (Wam) 1/8
sea salt 1/32
Shenf? 1/32
honey 1/8
Fresh beer 5/6

made as pills and people swallow them and drink beer 5/6

Another Treatment:

Wam grains (vegetable) ¼
Shenf 1/32
corn 1/3

It is finely grinded and drunk in one day.

Other :

sndh 1
civet 1
 oil 1
red natron 1
ox manfahah* 1

Make tablets and eat in one day.

N.B:
manfahah is the fourth part of the stomach of the cow animal, and generally resembles the human stomach.

Other:

sulkon ?* 1
Acorus
Carthamus
fruits bread
Mountain oil (petroleum?)
fresh beer 1
It is smoothly mixed, filtered, and eaten in one day.

N.B:
sulkoon is Red lead oxide

Other :

snfh? 1
red natron 1
civet 1

A tablet and eaten in one day.

Other :

Love Bjsu (a plant called Bjsu in Egyptian) 1/8
wine 1/3
Ameem? 1/3

Heated and drunk in four days.

Other :

corn beer 1
cumin 1
A plant called in Egyptian (Zeis)
sutah? 1
garlic 1
ashd? 1
fresh beer

Cook and eat in one day.

Other:

tamarind seed 1
milk 1
honey 1
sndh? 1
wine

Cooked, filtered and eaten in four days, it is prescribed for stomach aches.

Other:

sndh? 1
heaart Al-Masaa (small bird) 1
honey 1
wine 1
black nightshade 1
fresh beer 1

Make tablets and eat in one day.

Bind(Other For Treatment Worm Bind T.medioca-nellata)

peppermint 1
gmeem (plant) ? 1
noi (plant is called moi in egyptian)
ameem ? 1

cooked ,filtered and eaten in one day .

Other :

Ma'aa (dates) 1/16
g ?hzm 1/8
cyperus 1/16
Siwar? 1/64
Shenf? 1/32
fennel 5/6
Ameem? 1/3
latency 1/64
fresh beer 1

Cooked and filtered and eaten for four days.

Other :

colocynth (Handal) 1/8
Salukun (lead oxide) 1/6
dough with foam 5/6
white oil 1/8
fresh beer

It is cooked and eaten, and it kills the worm bind.

Other:

Juniper tubers 1/3
white oil 1/3

eaten in one day.

A Treatment To Repel The Tingling From The Body, That Is, To Remove The Pain From It:

1/3 . live beef 1/3
Frankinsence 1/64
Auf 1/8
Juniper beans 1/16
fresh bread 1/8
 fresh beer 1/3

Filter, cook and eat in four days.

Other: To Remove Tingles (I.e. Pains) From The Body:

garlic 1/8
Medicinal fruits?
Sahab (milk) 1/3
fresh beer 1/2

Filter, cook and eat in four days.

Other:

shamt 1/64
Medicinal fruit 1/8
acacia leaf 1/32
goose fat 1/16
Juniper tubers 1/16
fresh beer 1/3

Filter , cook and eat in four days.

Other:

flour 1/8
Hrror? (grapes: berries) 1/16

ashd? 1/8
fig 1/8
Frankinsence 1/64
latency 1/64
Juniper fruits 1/16
goose fat 1/16
fresh beer 1/3

Filter,cook and eat in four days.

Ahao * (To Remove Anemia From The Body):

exiled?* lapis lazuli
siwar? 1
nutmeg 1
sik?* 1
wax 1
civet 1

mix together and paint with it

Then do for him the recipes for defecation until it is removed from his stomach, which are:

sndh? 1
hop 1
eggplant 1
flour 1

grind and mixe one thing, makes four tablets, and the patient eat.

N.B:
Ahao *: translated as chlorosis CHOLORIS AGYPTIAGA
Exiled lapis lazuli: It is called in Egyptian, Anrsept. It was said that it is the stone of the philosophers, and it is believed that it transforms minerals into gold.

sik: Aromatic pills paste with water, paste with violet oil and musk, placed in a linen thread, dried, and then used.

For Egyptian Anemia Accompanied By Sluggishness (I.e., Heaviness) In The Body, Which Removes What Is Real In The Body:

dry myrrh 1/64
Frankinsence 1/64
lapis lazuli 1/64
Siwar? 1/64
Eggplant 1/32
Lead Rust 1/32
Myrtus 1/16
ghzm? 1/8

antimony 1/64
hop 1/8
sndh? 1/8
colocynth 1/8
honey 1/8
Water soaked carob 1/32

It is cooked and mixed together and eaten hot, as it is nice and tried.

To Remove The Anemia From The Body Or Cut It:

fig 1/32
sea salt 1/8
fresh bread 1/8
fresh beer 1/3
Cook, filter and eats in one day and then make:
sndh? 1/8
siram? 5/6
honey ¼
fresh beer 1/2
It is eaten in four days.

Servet (To Ward Off A Disease Called Servite):

Date flour 1/3
colocynth flour 1/3
A little mezze (the wine)
It is cooked in half a dna of water 1 and given hot to the man or the woman, so he cools his condition until recovery.

Ahau (To Ward Off Ahaw Disease, Which Is An Internal Ache):

ghzm? 1/3
colocynth powder (bitter melon) 1/3
sea salt ½
date honey 1/3
1/3 . oil
Ameem? 1/3
A little fresh beer

Cook and drink hot.

Ahau (Other: To Ward Off Disease Of The Stomach):

sweet myrrh 1
Siwar ?
Hbab Al Batia? 1
honey 1

Mix one thing and paint it.

Serfet (To Ward Off The Insidious Servite Disease, Which Is A Localized Disease):

Lettuce juice? 1
Salukon 1
tamarix seeds 1
natron 1
sea salt 1

It is made one thing and give it to him.

Okhdu (Other Than To Ward Off The Okhdu, I.e., The Twing

sindh? 1/8
garlic 1/16
fig 1/8
colocynth (Handal) 1/3
black nightshade(or wolfberry) 1/8
latency 1/64
Ameem? 1/32
goose fat 1/8

fresh beer 1/3

make one thing and give it to him.

Okhdo (Others To Remove The Twinge: Takedo)

dom 1/16
dates 1/3
sour beer 1/3
flour 1/8
wine 1/3
donkey milk 1

Cooked and filtered and eaten in four days.

Ukhdu (To Remove The Khudu, Okhdu, Or 'Aye', I.e. Fatal Weakness, Death In The Body Of A Man Or A Woman):

acacia leaf ½
Hatata? 1/3
fruit of acacia? 1/3
juniper leaf 1/3
hatata? 1/3
fruit? 1/3
ghzm? ¼
indigo ¼
A seed called taho? ½
wolf's bane (Aconitum) ¼
black nightshade ¼
peppermint ¼

Mixed and made eatable and eaten in four days.

Other: To Cut The Pain Oukhdo From The Abdomen:

wheat bread 1/3
Barley bread 1/3
Alberni fell"the best dates that fall ¼
Shanf? (which is the paste or rabbit ear) 1/8
Alberni flour ¼
lemon ¼
ghzm 1/8

Cooked, filtered and eaten in four days.

N.B:
Al-Birni: a type of yellow, round dates, and it is the finest dates.

Other:

The origins of cyperus 1/16
cyperus Boustany 1/16
cyperus 1/16
juniper berries
Brashan Daro? *1/16
gum 1/32
goose fat ¼
honey ¼
a little water

It is cooked and water is added to it and eaten in four days.

N.B:
brshan daro is Prostrate knotweed

(Hesbet Or...)

If you see a person with soft bloating and a crusty stomach below, then it is a stomach disease
If the swelling that is in his stomach does not find a way out or a way to get out of it (i.e. from the abdomen), then it is caused by a stubbornness in the abdomen.
If it doesn't mix, it's caused by the worm (I guess)
If it is not caused by the worm, then it is considered impossible to form a ball.
If he does not defecate, make him defecate recipes to get better now.

Notes:
Symptoms of stomach disease are:
 Soft tumor in the upper abdomen.
Solidification of any freezing caused by the presence of gases below the bulge.

If the previous two cases are present and are accompanied by constipation, then they are from stomach rot.
If all the mentioned symptoms are present and the constipation is continuous and complete, then it is caused by the presence of worms in the intestine or by a blockage in the lumen of the intestine by ossification of fecal material in it.
Given the clarity of the definition mentioned in the Egyptian text and its conformity with modern medicine, we can only acknowledge the ancient Egyptian thanks to his diagnosis of his previous thought in describing symptoms.

Ohau:other: To Remove The Groin (That Is, The Pain From The Abdomen) And To Cut Off A Disease That Affects The Abdomen Of Both Men And Women:

hot carob soaking ¼

bond? 1/8
Tamarind soaking 1/8
date soaking 1/8
goose fat 1/4
honey 1/4

One thing is made and eaten in one day.

The Principle Of Paints To Ward Off Disease (Ahao):

exiled? lapis lazuli
Milk
pure oil

Paint it for four days.

Another Paint:

acacia leaf
siwar?
exiled? lapis lazuli
washing stuff?
red natron
honey
oil

paint with.

Another Paint:

shnaf?
donkey head
nutmeg
a plant called septate
Carthamus
Maika Betty (Basisa)*
faq?(cooked oil)
pure oil
paint with

N.B:
Bsisa is a typical Mediterranean food, based on flour of roasted barley which dates back to Roman times. Bsisa is a variety of

mixtures of roasted cereals ground with fenugreek and aniseed and cumin and sugar. This kind of food is known throughout Tunisia and Libya.

Other Paint:

colocynth
bean flour
Carthamus
Siwar?
faq(cooked oil)
pure oil

Paint it for four days.

Other Paint:

sndh? grip
donkey hoof
Fresh cream
pure oil.

Paint it for four days.

Other Paint:

Hot sandy barley bread
Aat(a plant called in Egyptian Aat)
Dom hot
exiled? lapis lazuli
The milk of a woman who gave birth to a male
Fresh faq (Hot Oil)

Paint it for seven days.

Other:

nutmeg
Abit? (basil)
A plant called in Egyptian (Septet)
cool red sycamore
khat paper
pure oil
olive oil

Paint it seven days.

Other Paint:

Maikah? (Basisa) home made
flax seed
Curcuma
sk?
poppy seeds
cumin
wax
oil
faq(cooked oil)
The milk of a woman who gave birth to a male

Paint it eleven days.

Other Paint:

(Chefshouf) Basbasa*
lettuce seed
 sk?

colocynth
exiled? lapis lazuli
Curcuma
dry myrrh
sweet myrrh

Mix one thing and paint it.

N.B:
bsbasa : nutmeg

Another Treatment To Ward Off Ahaw Disease And To Ward Off Aches And Pains:

bull gland 5/6
sea salt 1/8
honey 1/32
½ . water

Mix one thing and paint it.

Another Remedy: To Ward Off The Disease (Ahaw) And To Ward Off The Twinge, I.e. The Pain:

bull gland 5/6
sea salt 1/8
honey 1/32
½ . water

Mix one thing and paint it.

Auhau (To Ward Off Auhau From Human Organs):

white oil 1
sea buffalo fat ? 1
honey
ghzm?
Remaining Karsana * 1
wax 1
Myrtle 1
Siwar?? 1
garlic 1
nutmeg 1
civet 1

Mix one thing and paint it for four days.

N.B:
karsana: Vicia ervilia, commonly known as ervil[1] or bitter

vetch, is an ancient grain legume crop of the Mediterranean region.

Another Paint To Remove The "Awha" From Every Human Organ:

sweet myrrh 1
Siwar? 1
oil 1
colocynth 1
Maidenhair fern 1
antimony 1
Hbab al-Batiyah (pottery utensils)
honey 1

Mix one thing and paint it.

(Ohau) And (Okhdo) To Remove The Aches Of The Oohau And Take Out The Pains: Okhdo:

ox gall 1
sea salt 1
honey 1

Mix one thing and paint it.

(Al-Ohaw) "Another Paint To Remove The Ouhau From Every Part Of The Human Body."

sndh?
oil

paint with.

Serft ::Servet

Other To Prevent Disease Called Servet

oil 5/6
siete?(A crushed plant called Saye)t 1 .
sea salt 1
Oil 1 (love is called oil)

natron 1

It is finely grinded and mixed as one thing and applied to the organs.

Al-Awhaw:

oil 1
Aegilops
sea salt 1
Saiete (plant called saiete) 1
natron 1

is put on it.

Okhdo (Others To Remove The Sharp Pains And Okhdo):

poppy 1
lead oxide 1
lead rust 1
honey 1
sk? 1
doum 1
soggy?
sannan stone? 1
fragrance 1
grease 1

Make one thing and put it on.

Mouth Okhdu(Other To Remove The Pain Okhdu From Mouth):

ghzm? 1/8
garlic 1/8
am ? 1/16
Poppy seeds 1/8
Juniper berries 1/16
flour 1/8
Medicinal fruits 1/16
Lead Rust 1/32
shamt? 1/64
Sycamore fruits 1/8
am seed? (DNA) 1

Mix with water, filter and gargle with it for four days.

Okhdu "Other To Remove Pain Okhdu"

A paint made of castor bean is applied to the patient with a fracture with pus in it. The existing pain leaves the organs as if there was nothing in it.
And its smell is removed by the paint, as before, within a period of ten days: by applying it in the morning, it will remove it.
Tried thousands of thousands of times.

Okhdu "Other To Remove The Pain, Okhdu":

tortoise pagha? 1
natron 1
fresh Fak(oil) 1
civet? 1
Mix one thing and heat and paint it.

Other :To Remove The Peak Of Pain (I.e. Its Bout):

fig 1/8
wheat bread 1/32
Medicinal fruit 1/8
Lead Rust 1/32
water 1/3

Mixed and eaten in four days.

To Remove The Peak Of Pain (I.e. Its Bout):

shnf 1
heart of colocynth (Al-Handal) 1
Lead Rust 1/32

Myrrh (shasha) 1
acacia leaf 1
juniper leaf 1
cow milk 1

Cook together and drink in four days.

Okhdu (Others: To Relieve Pain, Okhdu):

wheat flour 1
Barley flour 1
Dom powder 1
khat? 1
honey 1

is placed on it.

Medicine To Treat The Abdomen And Treat The Anus:

milk ¾
1/8 . goose fat
carob powder 1/3
sindh? ¼
black nightshade ¼

Filter and eat in one day.

Other:

flour 1/3
Barley flour ¼
Date powder ¼
honey 1/16
sindh? ¼
1/8 . goose fat

Filter and eat in one day.

Other :

1/16 . goose fat
honey 1/16
sindh? ¼
fresh bread ¼

Filter and eat in one day.

Other :

colocynth water 1/2
honey 1/8

Filter and eat in four days.

Other :

wine 1/3
honey 1/32
sindh? 1/8
colocynth water ¼
sandy bread dough 1/3
¼ . goose fat

it is cooked and made sandy bread for eating everyday and drink frothy beer on it.

Other :

sndh? 1/8
Fresh beer 1/4
honey 1/16
Frankinsence 1/64
Juniper fruits 1/16
black nightshade 1/3
fig 1/8

Water is added to it, filtered and eaten every day.

"Al-A'i" Other Than It To Remove Aia (I.e., Weakness) From The Human Being, Remove Twinge, Ward Off Pain That Afflicts Man, And Treat Anus:

ghzm ? 1/8
Juniper fruits 1/16
honey 1/32
fresh beer 1/2

Filter and eat in four days.

Inflammation Of The Anus And Bladder With Gas (Or: A Treatment To Remove Inflammation From The Anus And From The Bladder, Which Causes Many Gases Without The Person Knowing):

lettuce 1
salt 1
watermelon 1

honey 1
made one thing and makes pills that are inserted into the anus.*

N.B:
suppository

Others For Cooling The Anus (Perhaps Hemorrhoids):

(Khabr or) 1 "seeds of plant called Khbror"
Borshan Daro (Prostrate knotweed) 1
Juniper fruits 1
frankinsence 1
lead rust 1
Plantago 1
cumin 1
honey 1
myrrh 1
Cinnamomum

Made as a pill placed in the anus.

Anal Pain (Others For Anal Pain Relief)

fig 1
sea salt 1
frankinsence 1
cow horn 1

Make a pill and put it in the anus.

To Remove Anal Pain:

Ibex fat 1
cumin 1

Make a pill and put it in the anus.

Anal Cooling Treatment:

faq (cooked oil) 1
colocynth water 1
oil 1
honey 1/3

Injected into the anus.

Other: A Remedy To Soften The Anus (I.e. Soothe It):

Frankinsence 1
Sahwat? 1 "a plant called Sahwat" in Egyptian.
poppy seeds 1
Juniper 1
cumin 1
antimony 1
colocynth 1
Agma (plural of Jamim, a name for a plant)?* 1
Faaq (cooked oil) 1
fat 1
liniment 1
sea salt 1

It is grinded soft and a suppository is made and placed in the anus for four days.

N.B:
grass

Fistula (Others For Anal Wound: Perhaps Fistula):

myrrh 1
Frankinsence 1

cyperus from garden 1
beach salt 1
Turmeric 1
coriander 1
oil 1
salt 1

It is cooked together and placed in a rag and placed on the anus.

Another Treatment:

Goose egg (called roe) 1
Turb egg (i.e a type of geese) 1

It is placed in the anus.

Anal Treatment:

milk 1/3
goose fat 1/8
carob powder 1/4
sindah ? 1/4
black nightshade 1/4

Filter and eat in one day.

Other :

Barley flour 1/4
Date powder 1/4
wheat flour 1/4
honey 1/16
sindah? 1/4
fat 1/8

It is made one thing and eat it in one day.

Other :

goose fat 1/16
honey 1/16
¼sindah ? 1/4
fresh bread 1/4

eaten in one day.

Other :

colocynth water 1
honey 1/8

Drink in four days.

Another Treatment:

wine 1/3
honey 1/32
sindah? 1/8
colocynth water (bitter melon) 1/4
BBQ dough (name for the ball) 1/4
goose fat 1/4

cooked and made as a ball and is eaten every day with   frothy beer.

Other:

sindah? 1/8
fresh beer 1/4
honey 1/16
Frankinsence 1/64
Juniper fruits 1/16
black nightshade 1/3
fig 1/8
Medicinal fruit 1/8
Add water to it and eat it in four days.

A Treatment To Keep Burning And Pain Away From The Anus, And Twingle Of Legs:

heart of colocynth (Al-Handal) 1/32
fresh bread 1/8
wax 1/16
goose fat 1/8
water 1/3

Mixed with water and eaten in four days.

To Remove Heartburn From The Anus:

myrrh 1
Ayohu 1 (a plant called Ayohu in Egyptian)
soggy 1
Prostrate knotweed 1
ghzm? 1
Rakkarak (saffron) 1
lead rust 1

Sycamore Origins 1
Haplophyllum tuberculatum 1
impure dates 1

It is cooked, mixed and eaten by a man or woman who is suffering from inflammation.

To Remove Anal Inflammation:

bean flour* 1
colocynth powder (bitter melon) 1
myrrh 1
hdm? (incense) 1
antimony 1

Make a suppository and put it in the anus.

N.B:
fava beans .

Physician's Prescription:

Atto? 1/64 (a plant called atto)
wine 1/3
Fat bull gall 1/2
sarkhon ?* 5/6
honey

Filter and inject into the anus.

N.B:
most close translation is Tarragon

Other :

Ox gall bladder 1/3
Hot milk 5/6
honey 1/3
Mahawi? (a drink called Mahawi)

Filter and inject into the anus in one day.

Other:

colocynth (yellow melon) 1
Aconitum 1
Water

Injected into the anus.

Other :

colocynth water 1
acacia leaf 1
buckthorn leaf 1
Muhwai drink?

Injected into the anus.

Other: For Anal Cooling:

colocynth powder (bitter melon) 1/32
ruta 1/32
honey ¼
water 1/3

Filter and eat in four days.

Other: To Soften The Vessels Of The Anus:

fat 1/64
acacia leaf 1/64

bandage it.

Other: To Heal The Sore Anus:

cow horn 1
1 piece of dry Liniment
wine scum(residual)

It is made suppository for a man or woman.

Another Suppository To Cool The Anus:

Myrrh (shasha) 1
colocynth powder 1
wine scum 1
Khabrur? 1 (Love is called Khabrur)
sea salt 1
Barley flour 1
Date powder 1
honey 1

It is made as suppository and is put in the anus.

Other: To Soften The Anus And Soften The Peritoneum:

fave bean flour 1
natron 1
mix with myyrh 1
And poppies from the town of (Masau)? 2
Adiantum 1
And juniper beans 1
and frankinsence 1
And colocynth powder (bitter melon) 1
and cumin 1
and honey 1
Then they are applied together and mixed with honey and made into a suppository and placed in the anus.

To Remove Magic From The Body:

The heart of the pigeon? 1
Heart of Azeet? 1
Frankinsence 1
sindah? 1
fresh beer

Mix it together and drink it.

Other :

Take from a plant (Amdaa)? dana * that is kept in the dew, and a person drinks it with a dose of water every day for four days.

N.B:
dns is a measure.

To Remove Magic From The Body Of A Man Or A Woman:

A plant called (Zeiss)? 1
Adiantum 1
bee honey 1
natron

Mixed together and eaten by a man or a woman.

To Remove Magic And Holy Deadly Aia? (I.e., Weakness) That Afflicts The Human Body:

cyperus buds 1/8
myrrh (shasha) 1/8
acacia asak seeds 1/64
lettuce 1/64
It is made as a powder and put on beer and the patient drinks it before bedtime.

Other:

Date powder is placed on the fat and then placed on the Shob? (i.e honey) is placed over the fire and added to it (Sarkhon?) and the stomach aching woman eats it .

Other:

lettuce 1/64
Sunflower seeds 1/16
acacia asak 1/64
coriander 1/8

Cook together and eat before sleep.

Other:

Sunflower 1/16
myrrh (shasha) 1/8
Cassia fistula 1/14 *
honey 5/6

Mixed together and eaten before sleep.

N.B:
 Note from the writer: I doubt the ratio is 1/64

Other :

grape 1/8
pie 1/16
sunflower 1/8
honey 1/16
myrrh (shasha) 1/16

It is grirnded and eaten before bed.

Other:

Lemon 1/16
Aconitum 1/16
Adiantum 1/16
doum 1/3
ghzm? 1/8
honey 1/3

Eat before sleep.

Other :

lettuce 1/64
coriander 1/16
doum 1/16
myrrh (shasha) 1/8
Sunflower 1/16
Cook with honey 5/6

And women eat it before sleeping.

Peritonitis:

Treatment to remove peritonitis:
doum 1
roasted barley 1
wheat flour? 1
Barley flour 1
khat? 1
honey 1
It is placed in the lower abdomen (i.e. on the peritoneum)

Other:

fig 1
cumin 1
carob powder 1
honey 1
beer foam 1

poultice it on the lower abdomen.

Other :

Juniper tubers 1
Frankinsence 1
ashd? 1
dates 1
oil 1

siram? 1

poultice it on the lower abdomen.

Other :

carob powder 1
honey 1
oil 1
peppermint 1
Khat 1

poultice it on the lower abdomen.

Other :

Pieces of flax roots 1
dough

It is placed on the lower abdomen of the person in pain

Other :

Grease the head by the amount of a bowl
It is placed on the lower abdomen.

Other :

Mix with Myrrh and placed on the lower abdomen.

Death (To Ward Off Death From The Human Body) "Which Is, To Protect The Human Body From A Fatal Disease":

acacia asak seeds 1
turmeric seeds 1
Juniper tubers 1
Heart and wazet? (a plant called Wazit) 1
Myrrh (shasha) 1

It is mixed softly and person eat it with honey.

Medication To Treat The Surface Of The Body:

colocynth (Handal) 1/16
Cumin 1/4
wine

Cook and eat in four days.

Other :

grinded barley 1/4
cyperus
Frankinsence 1/32
The heart of colocynth 1/32

Wata'a Sycamore (bread) 1/32
Juniper tubers 1/32
garlic 1/8

It is eaten in four days.

The Large Intestine (To Treat The Surface Of The Body And To Ward Off All Pain From The Abdomen, And To Treat The Large Intestine)

foamy fresh beer
colocynth 1/2
Put it in a bowl, it is praised against death..
Mix it with foam and heat it any time and drink a hna* of it every day.

N.B:

measure

To Ward Off The Burning Twinges From The Body:

fig 1
fist of grapes 1
(ashad?) 1
Juniper tubers 1
Frankinsence 1
shmt? 1
cumin 1
wati'a (bread) of dates 1
fresh beer

Cooked and filtered and eaten in four days.

Other For Diseases Of The Body:

acacia leaves 1/8
fresh beer 1/3

They are cooked, kept in the dew, filtered and eaten for four days.

The Principle Of Drugs That Make The Stomach Accept Bread:

fat meat 1/6
midad? 1/32
fig 1/8
Juniper tubers 1/16
Frankinsence 1/64
cumin 1/64
garlic 1/16
goose fat 1/8
grape 1/8
milk cream 1/3
Fresh beer 5/6

to drink .

Other :

fresh beer 1/3
Sakhfa (back fat) 1/3
milk cream 1/3
Date powder 1/8
wheat flour 1/8
Juniper tubers 1/16
frankinsence 1/64
shmt? 1/64
black nightshade 1/8
fig 1/8
goose fat 1/8

Cooked and filtered and eaten in four days.

Other :

Shanf 1/32 (a plant called paste or rabbit's ear)
Fresh beer 5/6

Cooked and filtered and eaten in one day.

Other :

wine 5/6
wheat grain 1/8

It is kept all night in the dew, filtered and eaten in one day.

Other :

garlic 1/8
carob 1/8
Frankinsence 1/64
hnin? (transparent water) 1/8
Lead Rust 1/32
wine one dna

Cooked and filtered and eaten in four days.

Other :

dried bread in the fire 5/6
carob 1/4
golden shower(cassia fistula) 1/32
honey 1/32
water 1/2 dna

Filter and eat in four days.

Other:

dry bread 1/8
carob 1/8
honey 1/32
water 5/6

It is mixed, filtered and eaten in four days.

Other :

Fat meat 1/16
wine 1/3
black nightshade 1/16
fig 1/16
Turmeric 1/11
Fresh beer a third of dna*

Cooked and filtered and eaten in four days.

N.B:
dna is a measure

Other:

waei'a? (bread) 1/8
Hakn? (bread called Hakan) 1/8
heart of dates 1/8
honey 1/32
wine 1/3

Cooked and filtered and eaten in one day.

Other : To Make The Stomach Accept Bread:

fig 1/8
carob 1/8
Frankinsence 1/32
heart of dates 1/32
onion 1/32
Fresh beer 5/6
fat meat 1/4
willow 1/8

Cooked and filtered and eaten in four days.

To Remove Bloating From The Body:

fig 1/8
ashd? 1/8
black nightshade 1/16
cumin 1/64
acacia leaf 1/32
midad ? 1/64
Peppermint 1/32
hop 1/8
fresh beer
It is kept in open air and eaten for four days.

Diarrhea:(Medication To Remove Tuhar?, Which Is Diarrhoea):

colocynth (Handal) mixed with honey and the patient drinks it with beer.

"This is the book of healing for every disease..

May Isis heal me,

Like she cured Horus of every disease happend to him from set when he killed his father Osiris.

O Isis,
You are the great witch
heal me
And save me me from every hateful, bad, and devilish thing..
And from seizering diseases
And the deadly and malignant diseases of all kinds that happen to me
As you rescued and saved your son, Horus

As I entered in the fire and came out of the water . so,
Is it possible that I will not fall into that evil today, by saying:" I am young and pitiful " ?

Oh Ra, you are the one who read this determination on your body
O Osiris, you are worshipped for your reverence
Ra recites for his bod
And Osiris is worshiped in honor of him
Come on, save me from every corrupt, bad, or demonic thing..
and from the types of malignant fevers that kill."

• To the extent that there are chapters of these incantations, it is said as many as possible as many thousands times as possible.

REFRENCES

References

1. WEKIPEDIA
2. ^ Jouanna, Jacques; Allies, Neil (2012), "Egyptian Medicine and Greek Medicine", Greek Medicine from Hippocrates to Galen, Brill, pp. 3–20, JSTOR 10.1163/j.ctt1w76vxr.6
3. ^ Said, Galal Zaki (17 November 2013). "Orthopaedics in the dawn of civilisation, practices in ancient Egypt". International Orthopaedics. 38 (4): 905–909. doi:10.1007/s00264-013-2183-z. ISSN 0341-2695. PMC 3971265. PMID 24240438.
4. ^ "Edwin Smith papyrus (Egyptian medical book)". Encyclopedia Britannica (Online ed.). Retrieved 1 January 2016.
5. ^ Arab, Sameh M. "Medicine in Ancient Egypt – Part 1". Arab World Books. Retrieved 18 November 2011.
6. ^ Fagan, Brian M. (2004). The Seventy Great Inventions of the Ancient World. Thames & Hudson. ISBN 978-0-50005130-6.
7. ^ WEINBERGER, B. (1946). FURTHER EVIDENCE THAT DENTISTRY WAS PRACTICED IN ANCIENT EGYPT, PHOENICIA AND GREECE. Bulletin of the History of Medicine,20(2), 188–195. Retrieved from http://www.jstor.org/stable/44441040
8. ^ Jump up to:a b DAWSON, W. (1927). THE BEGINNINGS OF MEDICINE: MEDICINE AND SURGERY IN ANCIENT EGYPT. Science Progress in the Twentieth Century (1919-1933), 22(86), 275–284. Retrieved from http://www.jstor.org/stable/43430010
9. ^ Griffith, F. Ll. (1898). The Petrie Papyri: Hieratic Papyri from Kahun and Gurob. London: Bernard Quaritch. (Please note the book pages run from back to front.)
10. ^ Bynum, W. F.; Hardy, Anne; Jacyna, Stephen; Lawrence, Christopher; Tansey, E.M. (2006). "The Rise of Science in Medicine, 1850–1913". The Western Medical Tradition: 1800-2000. Cambridge University Press. pp. 198–199. ISBN 978-0-521-47565-5.

11. ^ Dollinger, André. "The Kahun Gynaecological Papyrus". An introduction to the history and culture of Pharaonic Egypt. Kibbutz Reshafim. Retrieved 21 April 2012.
12. ^ Jump up to:a b c d e Dollinger, André (December 2002). "Ancient Egyptian Medicine". An introduction to the history and culture of Pharaonic Egypt. Kibbutz Reshafim.
13. ^ Jump up to:a b Breasted, James Henry (1930). The Edwin Smith Papyrus. Chicago, Illinois: The University of Chicago Press.
14. ^ Allen, James P (2005). The Art of Medicine in Ancient Egypt. New York: The Metropolitan Museum of Art. ISBN 978-0-300-10728-9.
15. ^ Jump up to:a b Bryan, Cyril (1932). The Ebers Papyrus. New York: D. Appleton and Company.
16. ^ Jump up to:a b c d Nunn, John F. (1996). Ancient Egyptian Medicine. Transactions of the Medical Society of London. 113. Norman, Oklahoma: University of Oklahoma Press. pp. 57–68. ISBN 978-0-8061-2831-3. PMID 10326089.
17. ^ Ritner, Robert K. (April 2000). "Innovations and Adaptations in Ancient Egyptian Medicine". Journal of Near Eastern Studies. 59(2): 107–117. doi:10.1086/468799. JSTOR 545610. PMID 16468204. S2CID 39263523.
18. ^ Dollinger, André. "Herbal Medicine". An introduction to the history and culture of Pharaonic Egypt. Kibbutz Reshafim. Retrieved 9 October 2015.
19. ^ Parkins, Michael D.; Szekrenyes, J. (March 2001). "Pharmacological Practices of Ancient Egypt" (PDF). Proceedings of the 10th Annual History of Medicine Days. Calgary, Alberta, Canada: The University of Calgary. pp. 5–11.
20. ^ "What progress did the Egyptians make in medical knowledge?". Medicine Through Time: Model Questions and Answers. Passmores Academy. Archived from the original on 1 May 2008. Retrieved 1 January 2016.
21. ^ Magner, Lois (1992). A History of Medicine. Boca Raton, Florida: CRC Press. p. 31. ISBN 978-0-8247-8673-1.
22. ^ Stiefel, Marc; Shaner, Arlene; Schaefer, Steven D. (February

2006). "The Edwin Smith Papyrus: The Birth of Analytical Thinking in Medicine and Otolaryngology". The Laryngoscope. 116 (2): 182–188. doi:10.1097/01.mlg.0000191461.08542.a3. ISSN 0023-852X. PMID 16467701. S2CID 35256503.

23. ^ El-Aref, Nevine (December 2006). "Too big for a coffin". Al-Ahram Weekly. Cairo, Egypt: Al-Ahram. Archived from the originalon 18 November 2014. Retrieved 1 January 2016.

24. ^ Hawass, Zahi (2003). "The tomb of the physician Qar". Hidden Treasures of the Egyptian Museum: One Hundred Masterpieces from the Centennial Exhibition (Supreme Council of Antiquities ed.). Cairo, Egypt: American University in Cairo Press. p. xx. ISBN 978-977424778-1.

25. ^ Lauer, Jean Philippe (3 January 2013). "Imhoteb Museum". Egypt Tourism News. Egypt Tourism Board. Retrieved 1 January2016.

26. ^ Jackson, Russell (6 December 2006). "Mummy of ancient doctor comes to light". The Scotsman. Edinburgh. Retrieved 24 March2011.

27. ^ Greiner, Ryan (2001). "Ancient Egyptian Medicine". Creighton University Virtual Museums. Creighton University. Retrieved 2 April 2011.

28. ^ Herodotus (25 February 2006) [First published 1890]. An Account of Egypt (from The History of Herodotus Translated into English, Vol. I, Pages 115–208). Translated by Macaulay, G. C. Project Gutenberg.

29. ^ Jump up to:a b Arab, Sameh M. "Medicine in Ancient Egypt – Part 3". Arab World Books. Retrieved 18 November 2011.

30. ^ "Medicine in Ancient Egypt", SpringerReference, Springer-Verlag, 2011, doi:10.1007/springerreference_78530

31. ^ Gordan, Andrew H.; Shwabe, Calvin W. (2004). The Quick and the Dead: Biomedical Theory in Ancient Egypt. Egyptological Memoirs. Leiden: Brill Academic Publishers. p. 154. ISBN 978-90-04-12391-5.

32. ^ Grajetzki, Wolfram; Quirke, Stephen (2003). "Knowledge and production: the House of Life". Digital Egypt for Universities. University College London. Retrieved 18 November 2011.

33. ^ Bareš, Ladislav (2005). "The Shaft Tomb of Udjahorresnet". Czech Institute of Egyptology. Charles University in Prague. Retrieved 1 January 2016.

34. ^ Wood, Gemma Ellen (4 July 2012). "Dispelling the myth – Herodotus, Cambyses, and Egyptian religion #1". The Egyptiana Emporium. Retrieved 1 January 2016.

35. ^ Jump up to:a b c Agut-Labordère, Damien (2013). "The Saite Period: The Emergence of a Mediterranean Power". Ancient Egyptian Administration. Handbook of Oriental Studies. Leiden: Brill Academic Publishers. pp. 965–1027. ISBN 978-90-04-24952-3.

36. ^ "Wedjahor-Resne". Livius.org. Jona Lendering. 22 August 2015. Retrieved 1 January 2016.

37. ^ Fonahn, Adolf (1 January 1909). "Der altägyptische Arzt Iwti". Archiv für Geschichte der Medizin. 2 (5): 375–378. JSTOR 20772830.

38. ^ Fonahn, Adolf (February 1909). "Der altägyptische Arzt Iwti". Archiv für Geschichte der Medizin (in German). 2 (5): 375–378. JSTOR 20772830

39. Marry, Austin (January 21, 2004). "Ancient Egyptian Medical Papyri". Ancient Egypt Fan. Eircom Limited. Retrieved 2007-10-24.

40. ^ "medicine, health and wellbeing". EgyptologyOnline.com. Archived from the original on March 30, 2010. Retrieved 2007-10-26.

41. ^ Worton, Michael; Wilson-Tagoe, Nana (2004). National Healths: Gender, Sexuality and Health in a Cross-Cultural Context. London: UCL Press/Cavendish Publishing. p. 192. ISBN 978-1-84472-017-0. LCCN 2005295595.

42. ^ "History of the Library: late Middle Kingdom manuscripts from a tomb under the Ramesseum". Digital Egypt for Universities. University College London. 2003. Retrieved 2007-10-26.

43. ^ DiPaolo, Anthony C. (November 12, 2009). "The Papyrus Page". Anthony's Egyptology & Archaeology. Osiris Designs. Retrieved 2007-10-24.

44. ^ Martin, Andrew J. (2005-07-27). "Academy Papyrus to be Exhibited at the Metropolitan Museum of Art" (Press release). The New York Academy of Medicine. Archived from the original on November 27, 2010. Retrieved 2008-08-12.

45. ^ Wilkins, Robert H. (March 1964). "Neurosurgical Classic-XVII (Edwin Smith Surgical Papyrus)". Journal of Neurosurgery. 21 (3): 240–244. doi:10.3171/jns.1964.21.3.0240. PMID 14127631. translation of 13 cases from Breasted, James Henry (1930) pertaining to injuries of the skull and spinal cord, with commentary.

46. ^ "A Brief History of Migraines". Migraine and Headaches. Archived from the original on December 6, 2008. Retrieved 2007-10-24.

47. ^ Hickey, Todd M.; O'Connell, Elisabeth (2003). "The Hearst Medical Papyrus". The Center for the Tebtunis Papyri). Bancroft Library, University of California, Berkeley. Retrieved 2007-10-25.

48. ^ Owen, Antoinette; Danzing, Rachel (1993). "The History and Treatment of the Papyrus Collection at The Brooklyn Museum". In Espinosa, Robert (ed.). The Book and Paper Group Annual, Volume 12, 1993. American Institute for Conservation of Historic and Artistic Works. ISSN 0887-8978. LCCN 87640038.

49. ^ Jump up to:a b Sadek, Ashraf Alexandre (January 2001). "Some Aspects of Medicine in Pharonic Egypt". 50.History of Medicine. Australian Academy of Medicine & Surgery.

51."RCP". Archived from the original on 2007-09-28. Retrieved 2009-09-05.

52.Sandstead, Harold H.; Wagner, Conrad (2002-06-01). "William J. Darby, 1913–2001". The Journal of Nutrition. 132 (6): 1103–1106. doi:10.1093/jn/132.6.1103. ISSN 0022-3166. PMID 12042417.

53. Alt, Howard L. (1964-06-01). "Blood Diseases". Archives of Internal Medicine. 113 (6): 925. doi:10.1001/archinte.1964.00280120125054. ISSN 0003-9926.

54."PROFILE". ambassadors.net. Retrieved 2017-10-27.
International Congress of the History of Medicine

Ear, Nose and Throat in Ancient Egypt

55. Paul life
"Biomedical | Library | Vanderbilt University". www.mc.vanderbilt.edu. Retrieved 2017-10-27.

56. Letter from Paul Ghalioungui to C.L. Gemmill
"Naturwissenschaften und Medizin". www.kv5.de. Retrieved 2017-10-27.

57. 2001, Franz-Andre Sondervorst, Chronique de SIHM

58. David, R. (2008). "Redirecting". Lancet. 372 (9652): 1802–3. doi:10.1016/S0140-6736(08)61749-3. PMID 19048654. S2CID 35822210.

59. Dr. Paul Ghalioungui (1982), "The West denies Ibn Al Nafis's contribution to the discovery of the circulation", Symposium on Ibn al-Nafis, Second International Conference on Islamic Medicine: Islamic Medical Organization, Kuwait (cf. The West denies Ibn Al Nafis's contribution to the discovery of the circulation Archived 2009-08-25 at the Wayback Machine, Encyclopedia of Islamic World)

60. Yehia El-Rakhawi interview at Al-Ahram weekly Journal Archived 2009-08-07 at the Wayback Machine

Egyptian Medicine by Carloe Reeves 1992

62. "FindArticles.com | CBSi". findarticles.com. Retrieved 2017-10-27.

IDEO Archived 2011-07-24 at the Wayback Machine

63. "Remy Motte, Antiquaire, spécialiste boiseries et parquets anciens". Archived from the original on 2009-09-03. Retrieved 2009-09-13.

64. IDEO Archived 2011-07-24 at the Wayback Machine

65. "piccione, hist330, course bibliography". spinner.cofc.edu. Retrieved 2017-10-27.

66. Ghalioungui, Paul (1987). The Ebers papyrus: A new English translation, commentaries and glossaries. Academy of Scientific Research and Technology. ASIN B0006ERXEG.

67. "Paul Ghalioungui Books - List of books by Paul Ghalioungui". www.allbookstores.com. Retrieved 2017-10-27.

68. IDEO Archived 2011-07-24 at the Wayback Machine

69. Ghalioungui, Paul (1983). La médecine des pharaons: Magie et science médicale dans l'Egypte ancienne (in French). Paris: R. Laffont. ISBN 9782221011799.

70. Ghalioungui, Paul (1983). The physicians of Pharonic Egypt. Al-Ahram Center for Scientific Translations. ASIN B0006YCXJG.

71. Ghalioungui, Paul (1983). The physicians of Pharaonic Egypt (First ed.). Mainz a.Rh: Available from the U.S. Dept. of Commerce, National Technical Information Service. ISBN 9783805306003.

72. "Books by National Library of Medicine U S". 2014-02-12. Archived from the original on 2014-02-12.

73. "Journal of the History of Medicine and Allied Sciences | Oxford Academic". OUP Academic. Retrieved 2017-10-27.

74. The Physicians Of Phanasonic Egypt book review by Raja Reddy, B.I.I.H.M.Vol.XIV(1-4) Archived 2009-04-10 at the Wayback Machine

75. "Islamic Medical Manuscripts : Catalogue - Commentaries 2". www.nlm.nih.gov. Retrieved 2017-10-27.

76. "Archived copy" (PDF). Archived from the original (PDF) on 2008-12-20. Retrieved 2009-09-06.

77. Ghalioungui, Paul (1979). Kul-- lā ta'kul (in Arabic). Cairo: Dār al-Ma'ārif. ISBN 9789772478088.

78. IDEO Archived 2011-07-24 at the Wayback Machine

79. IDEO Archived 2011-07-24 at the Wayback Machine

80. Food history

Ghalioungui, Paul (1973). The house of life;: Per ankh. Magic and medical science in ancient Egypt ([2. herz. druk] ed.). Amsterdam: B. M. Israel. ISBN 9789060780626.

81. Kinnaer, Jacques. "The Ancient Egypt Site". www.ancient-egypt.org. Retrieved 2017-10-27.

82. ABD AL-LATIF (AL-BAGHDADI) Maqalatann fi-l-Hawass wa Masa'il Tabi'iya, Kuwait, Government Press, 83. 1972; texte arabe édité par Ghalioungui Paul et Abdou Said Archived 2009-09-05 at the Wayback Machine

84. Ghalioungui, Paul (1965). Magic and Medical Science in Ancient Egypt (Reprint ed.). Barnes And Noble. ASIN B001TD8ZOU.

85 . Magic and Medical Science in Ancient Egypt Archived 2011-05-18 at the Wayback Machine

86 . "The Oldest Medical Books in the World | Ancient Medicine | World Research Foundation". www.wrf.org. Retrieved 2017-10-27.

87 . "Archived copy". Archived from the original on 2011-07-06. Retrieved 2009-09-13.

Amazon.com

88 . "AAMS - Australian Academy of Medicine and Surgery". www.aams.org.au. Retrieved 2017-10-27.

89 . Ghalioungui, Paul (1965). Health and healing in ancient Egypt,: A pictorial essay. Dar al-Maaref. ASIN B0006FF400.

AFTERWORD

the script was translated from arabic . the notes mentioned was by the author

AFTERWORD

for further explanation , discussion or new researches . please contact dr. Alaa at his email: dr.alaaeldinhamada@gmail.com

BOOKS BY THIS AUTHOR

The Heart: Ancient Egyptian Cardiology

ancient egyptian cardiology is the original prescriptions from different papyri . tracing the substances and breaking the spells and names .
this book is a seed for discoveries in the field of medicine .

UNTITLED